Slow Cooker Dessert Recipes

Healthy Recipes for Your Slow Cooker

By Simon Tibbs

Sommario

Introduction 7

Slow Cooker Dessert Recipes 9

Introduction

We know you are always searching for easier methods to prepare your meals. We additionally recognize you are possibly sick and tired of investing lengthy hrs in the kitchen area food preparation with a lot of pans and pots. Well, currently your search is over! We located the excellent kitchen device you can utilize from now on! We are discussing the Slow stove! These remarkable pots permit you to prepare several of the very best dishes ever with minimal initiative Slow-moving cookers prepare your meals easier and a lot much healthier! You do not require to be an expert in the kitchen to cook some of one of the most scrumptious, flavorful, textured and also rich recipes!

All you require is your Slow cooker as well as the ideal active ingredients!

This excellent cookbook you will find will show you just how to prepare the best slow-moving cooked dishes. It will reveal you that you can make some outstanding morning meals, lunch meals, side meals, chicken, meat and also fish meals. Lastly yet importantly, this cookbook offers you some straightforward and wonderful desserts.

Slow Cooker Dessert Recipes

Cinnamon Apples

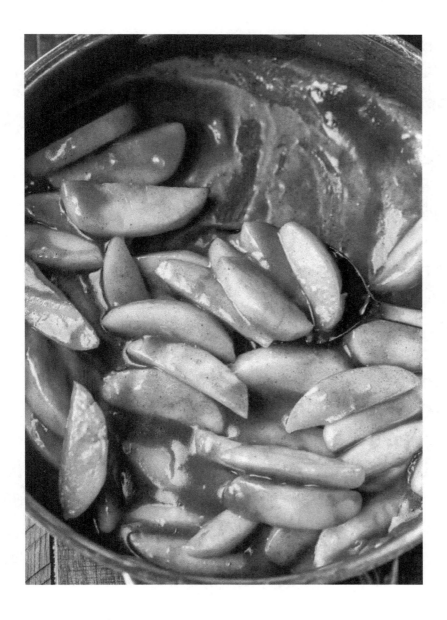

Preparation time: 10 minutes

Cooking time: 2 hours

Servings: 2

Ingredients:

- 2 tablespoons brown sugar

- 1 pound apples, cored and cut into wedges

- 1 tablespoon cinnamon powder

- 2 tablespoons walnuts, chopped

- A pinch of nutmeg, ground

- ½ tablespoon lemon juice

- ¼ cup water

- 2 apples, cored and tops cut off

Directions:

1. In your slow cooker, mix the apples with the sugar, cinnamon and the other ingredients, toss, put the lid on and cook on High for 2 hours.

2. Divide the mix between plates and serve.

Nutrition: calories 189, fat 4, fiber 7, carbs 19, protein 2

Peanut Butter Cake

Preparation time: 10 minutes

Cooking time: 2 hours and 30 minutes

Servings: 8

Ingredients:

- 1 cup sugar

- 1 cup flour

- 3 tablespoons cocoa powder+ ½ cup

- 1 and ½ teaspoons baking powder

- ½ cup milk

- 2 tablespoons vegetable oil

- 2 cups hot water

- 1 teaspoon vanilla extract

- ½ cup peanut butter

- Cooking spray

Directions:

1. In a bowl, mix half of the sugar with 3 tablespoons cocoa, flour, baking powder, oil, vanilla and milk, stir well and pour into your Slow cooker greased with cooking spray.

2. In another bowl, mix the rest of the sugar with the rest of the cocoa, peanut butter and hot water, stir well and pour over the batter in the slow cooker.

3. Cover slow cooker, cook on High for 2 hours and 30 minutes, slice cake and serve.

Nutrition: calories 242, fat 4, fiber 7, carbs 8, protein 4

Vanilla Pears

Preparation time: 10 minutes

Cooking time: 2 hours

Servings: 2

Ingredients:

- 2 tablespoons avocado oil

- 1 teaspoon vanilla extract

- 2 pears, cored and halved

- ½ tablespoon lime juice

- 1 tablespoon sugar

Directions:

1. In your slow cooker combine the pears with the sugar, oil and the other ingredients, toss, put the lid on and cook on High for 2 hours.

2. Divide between plates and serve.

Nutrition: calories 200, fat 4, fiber 6, carbs 16, protein 3

Blueberry Cake

Preparation time: 10 minutes

Cooking time: 1 hour

Servings: 6

Ingredients:

- ½ cup flour

- ¼ teaspoon baking powder

- ¼ teaspoon sugar

- ¼ cup blueberries

- 1/3 cup milk

- 1 teaspoon olive oil

- 1 teaspoon flaxseed, ground

- ½ teaspoon lemon zest, grated

- ¼ teaspoon vanilla extract

- ¼ teaspoon lemon extract

- Cooking spray

Directions:

1. In a bowl, mix flour with baking powder, sugar, blueberries, milk, oil, flaxseeds, lemon zest, vanilla extract and lemon extract and whisk well.

2. Spray your slow cooker with cooking spray, line it with parchment paper, pour cake batter, cover slow cooker, cook on High for 1 hour, leave the cake to cool down, slice and serve.

Nutrition: calories 200, fat 4, fiber 4, carbs 10, protein 4

Avocado Cake

Preparation time: 10 minutes

Cooking time: 2 hours

Servings: 2

Ingredients:

- ½ cup brown sugar

- 2 tablespoons coconut oil, melted

- 1 cup avocado, peeled and mashed

- ½ teaspoon vanilla extract

- 1 egg

- ½ teaspoon baking powder

- 1 cup almond flour

- ¼ cup almond milk

- Cooking spray

Directions:

1. In a bowl, mix the sugar with the oil, avocado and the other ingredients except the cooking spray and whisk well.

2. Grease your slow cooker with cooking spray, add the cake batter, spread, put the lid on and cook on High for 2 hours.

3. Leave the cake to cool down, slice and serve.

Nutrition: calories 300, fat 4, fiber 4, carbs 27, protein 4

Peach Pie

Preparation time: 10 minutes

Cooking time: 4 hours

Servings: 4

Ingredients:

- 4 cups peaches, peeled and sliced

- 1 cup sugar

- ½ teaspoon cinnamon powder

- 1 and ½ cups crackers, crushed

- ¼ teaspoon nutmeg, ground

- ½ cup milk

- 1 teaspoon vanilla extract

- Cooking spray

Directions:

1. In a bowl, mix peaches with half of the sugar and cinnamon and stir.

2. In another bowl, mix crackers with the rest of the sugar, nutmeg, milk and vanilla extract and stir.

3. Spray your Slow cooker with cooking spray, spread peaches on the bottom, add crackers mix, spread, cover and cook on Low for 4 hours.

4. Divide cobbler between plates and serve.

Nutrition: calories 212, fat 4, fiber 4, carbs 7, protein 3

Coconut Cream

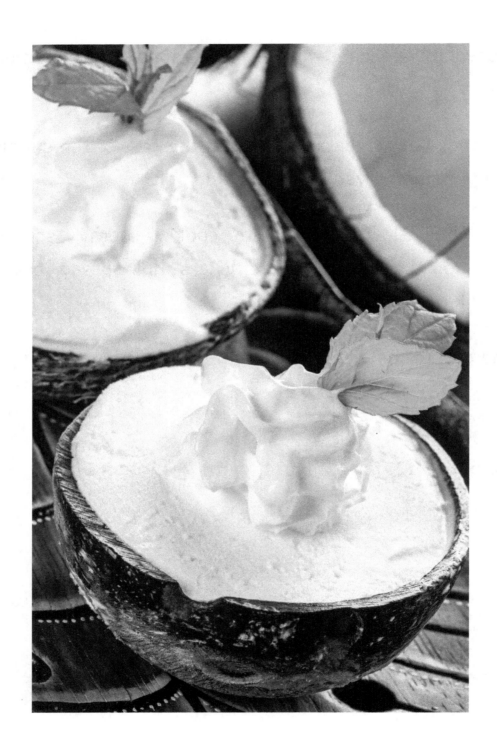

Preparation time: 10 minutes

Cooking time: 1 hour

Servings: 2

Ingredients:

- 2 ounces coconut cream

- 1 cup coconut milk

- ½ teaspoon almond extract

- 2 tablespoons sugar

Directions:

1. In your slow cooker, mix the cream with the milk and the other ingredients, whisk, put the lid on, cook on High for 1 hour, divide into bowls and serve cold.

Nutrition: calories 242, fat 12, fiber 6, carbs 9, protein 4

Sweet Strawberry Mix

Preparation time: 10 minutes

Cooking time: 3 hours

Servings: 10

Ingredients:

- 2 tablespoons lemon juice

- 2 pounds strawberries

- 4 cups sugar

- 1 teaspoon cinnamon powder

- 1 teaspoon vanilla extract

Directions:

1. In your Slow cooker, mix strawberries with sugar, lemon juice, cinnamon and vanilla, cover, cook on Low for 3 hours, divide into bowls and serve cold.

Nutrition: calories 100, fat 1, fiber 1, carbs 6, protein 2

Almond Rice Pudding

Preparation time: 10 minutes

Cooking time: 1 hour

Servings: 2

Ingredients:

- 2 tablespoons almonds, chopped

- 1 cup white rice

- 2 cups almond milk

- 1 tablespoon sugar

- 1 tablespoons maple syrup

- ¼ teaspoon cinnamon powder

- ¼ teaspoon ginger, grated

Directions:

1. In your slow cooker, mix the milk with the rice, sugar and the other ingredients, toss, put the lid on and cook on High for 1 hour.

2. Divide the pudding into bowls and serve cold

Nutrition: calories 205, fat 2, fiber 7, carbs 11, protein 4

Sweet Plums

Preparation time: 10 minutes

Cooking time: 3 hours

Servings: 6

Ingredients:

- 14 plums, halved

- 1 and ¼ cups sugar

- 1 teaspoon cinnamon powder

- ¼ cup water

Directions:

1. Put the plums in your Slow cooker, add sugar, cinnamon and water, stir, cover, cook on Low for 3 hours, divide into bowls and serve cold

Nutrition: calories 150, fat 2, fiber 1, carbs 5, protein 3

Cherry Bowls

Preparation time: 10 minutes

Cooking time: 1 hour

Servings: 2

Ingredients:

- 1 cup cherries, pitted

- 1 tablespoon sugar

- ½ cup red cherry juice

- 2 tablespoons maple syrup

Directions:

1. In your slow cooker, mix the cherries with the sugar and the other ingredients, toss gently, put the lid on, cook on High for 1 hour, divide into bowls and serve.

Nutrition: calories 200, fat 1, fiber 4, carbs 5, protein 2

Bananas and Sweet Sauce

Preparation time: 10 minutes

Cooking time: 2 hours

Servings: 4

Ingredients:

- Juice of ½ lemon

- 3 tablespoons agave nectar

- 1 tablespoon vegetable oil

- 4 bananas, peeled and sliced

- ½ teaspoon cardamom seeds

Directions:

1. Put the bananas in your Slow cooker, add agave nectar, lemon juice, oil and cardamom, cover, cook on Low for 2 hours, divide bananas between plates, drizzle agave sauce all over and serve.

Nutrition: calories 120, fat 1, fiber 2, carbs 8, protein 3

Berry Cream

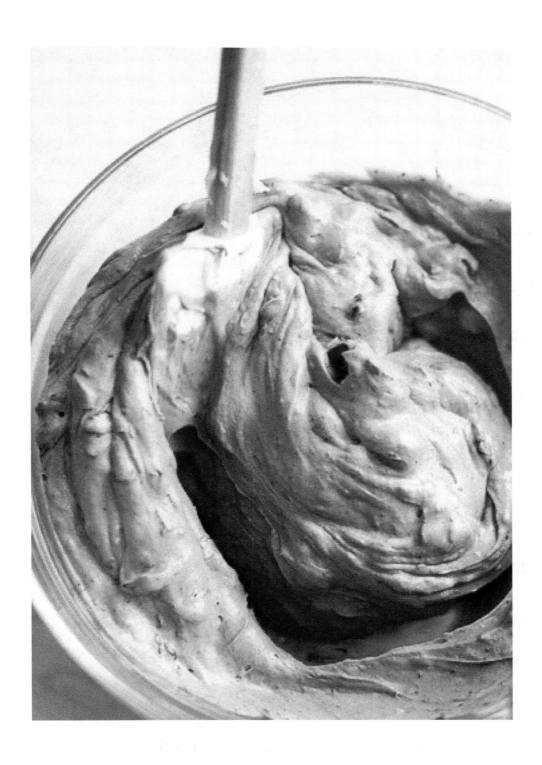

Preparation time: 10 minutes

Cooking time: 2 hours

Servings: 2

Ingredients:

- 2 tablespoons cashews, chopped

- 1 cup heavy cream

- ½ cup blueberries

- ½ cup maple syrup

- ½ tablespoon coconut oil, melted

Directions:

1. In your slow cooker, mix the cream with the berries and the other ingredients, whisk, put the lid on and cook on Low for 2 hours.

2. Divide the mix into bowls and serve cold.

Nutrition: calories 200, fat 3, fiber 5, carbs 12, protein 3

Orange Cake

Preparation time: 10 minutes

Cooking time: 5 hours

Servings: 4

Ingredients:

- Cooking spray

- 1 teaspoon baking powder

- 1 cup flour

- 1 cup sugar

- ½ teaspoon cinnamon powder

- 3 tablespoons vegetable oil

- ½ cup milk

- ½ cup pecans, chopped

- ¾ cup water

- ½ cup raisins

- ½ cup orange peel, grated

- ¾ cup orange juice

Directions:

1. In a bowl, mix flour with half of the sugar, baking powder, cinnamon, 2 tablespoons oil, milk, pecans and raisins, stir and pour this into your Slow cooker greased with cooking spray.

2. Heat up a small pan over medium heat, add water, orange juice, orange peel, the rest of the oil and the rest of the sugar, stir, bring to a boil, pour over the mix in the Slow cooker, cover and cook on Low for 5 hours.

3. Divide into dessert bowls and serve cold.

Nutrition: calories 182, fat 3, fiber 1, carbs 4, protein 3

Maple Pudding

Preparation time: 10 minutes

Cooking time: 1 hour

Servings: 2

Ingredients:

- ¼ cup cashew butter

- 1 tablespoon coconut oil, melted

- ½ cup white rice

- 1 cup almond milk

- 2 tablespoons lemon juice

- ½ teaspoon lemon zest, grated

- 1 tablespoon maple syrup

Directions:

1. In your slow cooker, mix the rice with the milk, coconut oil and the other ingredients, whisk, put the lid on and cook on High for 1 hour.

2. Divide into bowls and serve.

Nutrition: calories 202, fat 4, fiber 5, carbs 14, protein 1

Apples Stew

Preparation time: 10 minutes

Cooking time: 1 hour and 30 minutes

Servings: 5

Ingredients:

- 5 apples, tops cut off and cored

- 1/3 cup sugar

- ¼ cup pecans, chopped

- 2 teaspoons lemon zest, grated

- ½ teaspoon cinnamon powder

- 1 tablespoon lemon juice

- 1tablespoon vegetable oil

- ½ cup water

Directions:

1. Arrange apples in your Slow cooker, add sugar, pecans, lemon zest, cinnamon, lemon juice, coconut oil and water, toss, cover and cook on High for 1 hour and 30 minutes.

2. Divide apple stew between plates and serve.

Nutrition: calories 200, fat 1, fiber 2, carbs 6, protein 3

Chia and Orange Pudding

Preparation time: 10 minutes

Cooking time: 1 hour

Servings: 2

Ingredients:

- 1 tablespoon chia seeds

- ½ cup almond milk

- ½ cup oranges, peeled and cut into segments

- 1 tablespoon sugar

- ½ teaspoon cinnamon powder

- 1 tablespoon coconut oil, melted

- 2 tablespoons pecans, chopped

Directions:

1. In your slow cooker, mix the chia seeds with the almond milk, orange segments and the other ingredients, toss, put the lid on and cook on High for 1 hour.

2. Divide the pudding into bowls and serve cold.

Nutrition: calories 252, fat 3, fiber 3, carbs 7, protein 3

Pears and Sauce

Preparation time: 10 minutes

Cooking time: 4 hours

Servings: 4

Ingredients:

- 4 pears, peeled and cored

- 2 cups orange juice

- ¼ cup maple syrup

- 2 teaspoons cinnamon powder

- 1 tablespoon ginger, grated

Directions:

1. In your Slow cooker, mix pears with orange juice, maple syrup, cinnamon and ginger, cover and cook on Low for 4 hours.

2. Divide pears and sauce between plates and serve warm.

Nutrition: calories 210, fat 1, fiber 2, carbs 6, protein 4

Creamy Berries Mix

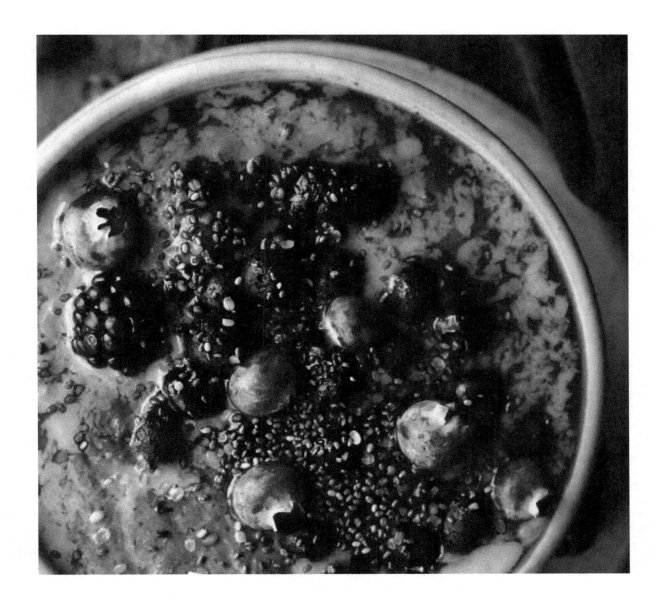

Preparation time: 10 minutes

Cooking time: 1 hour

Servings: 2

Ingredients:

- ½ teaspoon nutmeg, ground

- ½ teaspoon vanilla extract

- ½ cup blackberries

- ½ cup blueberries

- ¼ cup whipping cream

- 1 tablespoon sugar

- 2 tablespoons walnuts, chopped

Directions:

1. In your slow cooker, combine the berries with the cream and the other ingredients, toss gently, put the lid on, cook on High for 1 hour, divide into bowls, and serve.

Nutrition: calories 260, fat 3, fiber 2, carbs 14, protein 3

Vanilla Cookies

Preparation time: 10 minutes

Cooking time: 2 hours and 30 minutes

Servings: 12

Ingredients:

- 2 eggs

- ¼ cup vegetable oil

- 1 cup sugar

- ½ teaspoon vanilla extract

- 1 teaspoon baking powder

- 1 and ½ cups almond meal

- ½ cup almonds, chopped

Directions:

1. In a bowl, mix oil with sugar, vanilla extract and eggs and whisk.

2. Add baking powder, almond meal and almonds and stir well.

3. Line your slow cooker with parchment paper, spread cookie mix on the bottom of the slow cooker, cover and cook on Low for 2 hours and 30 minutes.

4. Leave cookie sheet to cool down, cut into medium pieces and serve.

Nutrition: calories 220, fat 2, fiber 1, carbs 3, protein 6

Apple Compote

Preparation time: 10 minutes

Cooking time: 1 hour

Servings: 2

Ingredients:

- 1 pound apples, cored and cut into wedges

- ½ cup water

- 1 tablespoon sugar

- 1 teaspoon vanilla extract

- ½ teaspoon almond extract

Directions:

1. In your slow cooker, mix the apples with the water and the other ingredients, toss, put the lid on and cook on High for 1 hour.

2. Divide into bowls and serve cold.

Nutrition: calories 203, fat 0, fiber 1, carbs 5, protein 4

Pumpkin Pie

Preparation time: 10 minutes

Cooking time: 2 hours and 20 minutes

Servings: 10

Ingredients:

- 1 and ½ teaspoons baking powder

- Cooking spray

- 1 cup pumpkin puree

- 2 cups flour

- ½ teaspoon baking soda

- 1 and ½ teaspoons cinnamon powder

- ¼ teaspoon ginger, grated

- 1 tablespoon vegetable oil

- 2 eggs

- 1 tablespoon vanilla extract

- 1/3 cup maple syrup

- 1 teaspoon lemon juice

Directions:

1. In a bowl, flour with baking powder, baking soda, cinnamon, ginger, eggs, oil, vanilla, pumpkin puree, maple syrup and lemon juice, stir and pour in your slow cooker greased with cooking spray and lined.

2. Cover slow cooker and cook on Low for 2 hours and 20 minutes.

3. Leave the cake to cool down, slice and serve.

Nutrition: calories 182, fat 3, fiber 2, carbs 10, protein 3

Plums Stew

Preparation time: 10 minutes

Cooking time: 1 hour

Servings: 2

Ingredients:

- 1 pound plums, pitted and halved

- ½ teaspoon nutmeg, ground

- 1 cup water

- 1 and ½ tablespoons sugar

- 1 tablespoon vanilla extract

Directions:

1. In your slow cooker, mix the plums with the water and the other ingredients, toss gently, put the lid on and cook on High for 1 hour.

2. Divide the mix into bowls and serve.

Nutrition: calories 200, fat 2, fiber 1, carbs 5, protein 4

Strawberries Marmalade

Preparation time: 10 minutes

Cooking time: 4 hours

Servings: 10

Ingredients:

- 32 ounces strawberries, chopped

- 2 pounds sugar

- Zest of 1 lemon, grated

- 4 ounces raisins

- 3 ounces water

Directions:

1. In your slow cooker, mix strawberries with coconut sugar, lemon zest, raisins and water, stir, cover and cook on High for 4 hours.

2. Divide into small jars and serve cold.

Nutrition: calories 140, fat 3, fiber 2, carbs 2, protein 1

Cinnamon Peach Mix

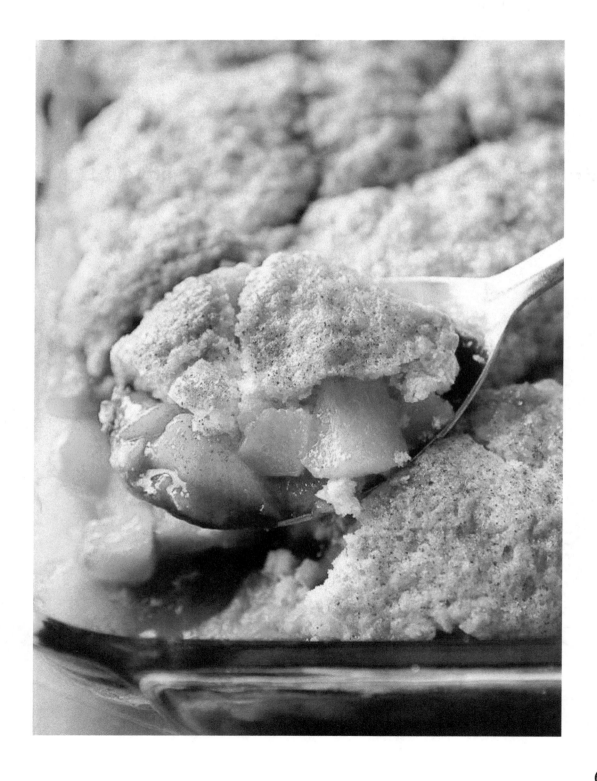

Preparation time: 10 minutes

Cooking time: 2 hours

Servings: 2

Ingredients:

- 2 cups peaches, peeled and halved

- 3 tablespoons sugar

- ½ teaspoon cinnamon powder

- ½ cup heavy cream

- 1 teaspoon vanilla extract

Directions:

5. In your slow cooker, mix the peaches with the sugar and the other ingredients, toss, put the lid on and cook on High for 2 hours.

6. Divide the mix into bowls and serve.

Nutrition: calories 212, fat 4, fiber 4, carbs 7, protein 3

Rhubarb Marmalade

Preparation time: 10 minutes

Cooking time: 3 hours

Servings: 8

Ingredients:

- 1/3 cup water

- 2 pounds rhubarb, chopped

- 2 pounds strawberries, chopped

- 1 cup sugar

- 1 tablespoon mint, chopped

Directions:

1. In your Slow cooker, mix water with rhubarb, strawberries, sugar and mint, stir, cover and cook on High for 3 hours.

2. Divide into cups and serve cold.

Nutrition: calories 100, fat 1, fiber 4, carbs 10, protein 2

Strawberry Cake

Preparation time: 10 minutes

Cooking time: 1 hour

Servings: 2

Ingredients:

- ¼ cup coconut flour

- ¼ teaspoon baking soda

- 1 tablespoon sugar

- ¼ cup strawberries, chopped

- ½ cup coconut milk

- 1 teaspoon butter, melted

- ½ teaspoon lemon zest, grated

- ¼ teaspoon vanilla extract

- Cooking spray

Directions:

3. In a bowl, mix the coconut flour with the baking soda, sugar and the other ingredients except the cooking spray and stir well.

4. Grease your slow cooker with the cooking spray, line it with parchment paper, pour the cake batter inside, put the lid on and cook on High for 1 hour.

5. Leave the cake to cool down, slice and serve.

Nutrition: calories 200, fat 4, fiber 4, carbs 10, protein 4

Sweet Potato Pudding

Preparation time: 10 minutes

Cooking time: 5 hours

Servings: 8

Ingredients:

- 1 cup water

- 1 tablespoon lemon peel, grated

- ½ cup sugar

- 3 sweet potatoes peeled and sliced

- ¼ cup butter

- ¼ cup maple syrup

- 1 cup pecans, chopped

Directions:

1. In your Slow cooker, mix water with lemon peel, sugar, potatoes, butter, maple syrup and pecans, stir, cover and cook on High for 5 hours.

2. Divide sweet potato pudding into bowls and serve cold.

Nutrition: calories 200, fat 4, fiber 3, carbs 10, protein 4

Ginger Pears Mix

Preparation time: 10 minutes

Cooking time: 2 hours

Servings: 2

Ingredients:

- 2 pears, peeled and cored

- 1 cup apple juice

- ½ tablespoon brown sugar

- 1 tablespoon ginger, grated

Directions:

1. In your slow cooker, mix the pears with the apple juice and the other ingredients, toss, put the lid on and cook on Low for 2 hour.

2. Divide the mix into bowls and serve warm.

Nutrition: calories 250, fat 1, fiber 2, carbs 12, protein 4

Cherry Jam

Preparation time: 10 minutes

Cooking time: 3 hours

Servings: 6

Ingredients:

- 2 tablespoons lemon juice

- 3 tablespoons gelatin

- 4 cups cherries, pitted

- 2 cups sugar

Directions:

1. In your Slow cooker, mix lemon juice with gelatin, cherries and coconut sugar, stir, cover and cook on High for 3 hours.

2. Divide into cups and serve cold.

Nutrition: calories 211, fat 3, fiber 1, carbs 3, protein 3

Raisin Cookies

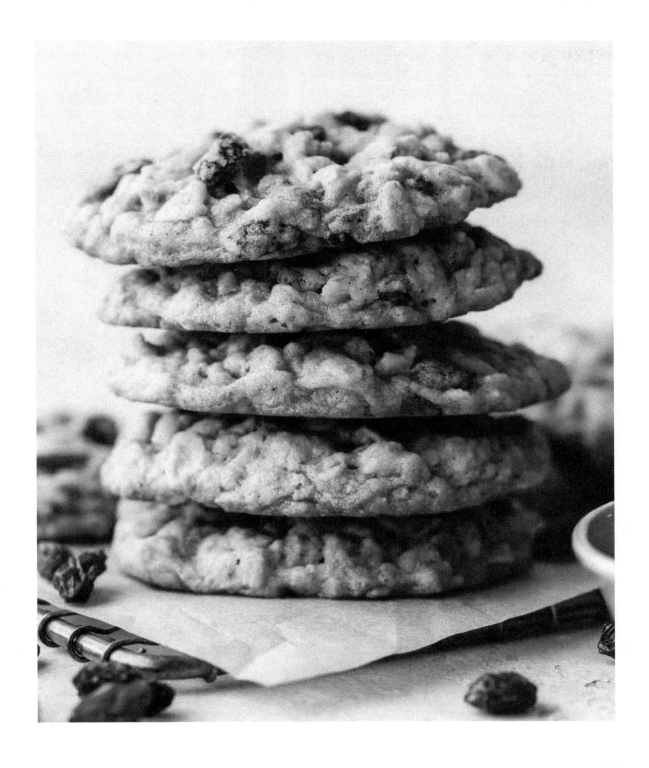

Preparation time: 10 minutes

Cooking time: 2 hours and 30 minutes

Servings: 2

Ingredients:

- 1 tablespoon coconut oil, melted

- 2 eggs, whisked

- ¼ cup brown sugar

- ½ cup raisins

- ¼ cup almond milk

- ¼ teaspoon vanilla extract

- ¼ teaspoon baking powder

- 1 cup almond flour

Directions:

1. In a bowl, mix the eggs with the raisins, almond milk and the other ingredients and whisk well.

2. Line your slow cooker with parchment paper, spread the cookie mix on the bottom of the pot, put the lid on, cook on Low for 2 hours and 30 minutes, leave aside to cool down, cut with a cookie cutter and serve.

Nutrition: calories 220, fat 2, fiber 1, carbs 6, protein 6

Sweet Cookies

Preparation time: 10 minutes

Cooking time: 2 hours and 30 minutes

Servings: 10

Ingredients:

- 1 egg white

- ¼ cup vegetable oil

- 1 cup sugar

- ½ teaspoon vanilla extract

- 1 teaspoon baking powder

- 1 and ½ cups almond meal

- ½ cup dark chocolate chips

Directions:

1. In a bowl, mix coconut oil with sugar, vanilla extract and egg white and beat well using your mixer.

2. Add baking powder and almond meal and stir well.

3. Fold in chocolate chips and stir gently.

4. Line your slow cooker with parchment paper and grease it.

5. Transfer cookie mix to your Slow cooker, press it on the bottom, cover and cook on low for 2 hours and 30 minutes.

6. Take cookie sheet out of the Slow cooker, cut in 10 bars and serve.

Nutrition: calories 220, fat 2, fiber 1, carbs 3, protein 6

Blueberries Jam

Preparation time: 10 minutes

Cooking time: 4 hours

Servings: 2

Ingredients:

- 2 cups blueberries

- ½ cup water

- ¼ pound sugar

- Zest of 1 lime

Directions:

1. In your slow cooker, combine the berries with the water and the other ingredients, toss, put the lid on and cook on High for 4 hours.

2. Divide into small jars and serve cold.

Nutrition: calories 250, fat 3, fiber 2, carbs 6, protein 1

Maple Pears

Preparation time: 10 minutes

Cooking time: 4 hours

Servings: 4

Ingredients:

- 4 pears, peeled and tops cut off and cored

- 5 cardamom pods

- 2 cups orange juice

- ¼ cup maple syrup

- 1 cinnamon stick

- 1-inch ginger, grated

Directions:

1. Put the pears in your Slow cooker, add cardamom, orange juice, maple syrup, cinnamon and ginger, cover and cook on Low for 4 hours.

2. Divide pears between plates and serve them with the sauce on top.

Nutrition: calories 200, fat 4, fiber 2, carbs 3, protein 4

Orange Bowls

Preparation time: 10 minutes

Cooking time: 3 hours

Servings: 2

Ingredients:

- ½ pound oranges, peeled and cut into segments

- 1 cup heavy cream

- ½ tablespoon almonds, chopped

- 1 tablespoon chia seeds

- 1 tablespoon sugar

Directions:

1. In your slow cooker, mix the oranges with the cream and the other ingredients, toss, put the lid on and cook on Low for 3 hours.

2. Divide into bowls and serve.

Nutrition: calories 170, fat 0, fiber 2, carbs 7, protein 4

Stuffed Apples

Preparation time: 10 minutes

Cooking time: 1 hour and 30 minutes

Servings: 5

Ingredients:

- 5 apples, tops cut off and cored

- 5 figs

- 1/3 cup sugar

- 1 teaspoon dried ginger

- ¼ cup pecans, chopped

- 2 teaspoons lemon zest, grated

- ¼ teaspoon nutmeg, ground

- ½ teaspoon cinnamon powder

- 1 tablespoon lemon juice

- 1tablespoon vegetable oil

- ½ cup water

Directions:

1. In a bowl, mix figs with sugar, ginger, pecans, lemon zest, nutmeg, cinnamon, oil and lemon juice, whisk really well, stuff your apples with this mix and put them in your Slow cooker.

2. Add the water, cover, cook on High for 1 hour and 30 minutes, divide between dessert plates and serve.

Nutrition: calories 200, fat 1, fiber 2, carbs 4, protein 7

Quinoa Pudding

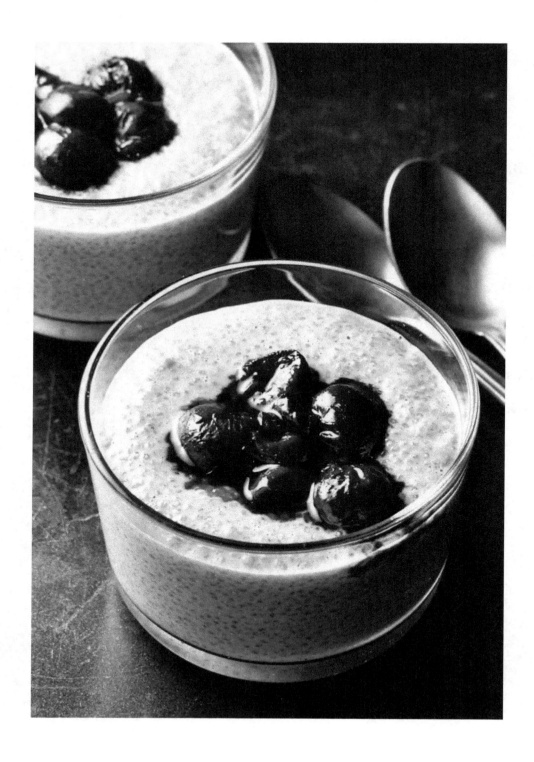

Preparation time: 10 minutes

Cooking time: 2 hours

Servings: 2

Ingredients:

- 1 cup quinoa

- 2 cups almond milk

- ½ cup sugar

- ½ tablespoon walnuts, chopped

- ½ tablespoon almonds, chopped

Directions:

1. In your slow cooker, mix the quinoa with the milk and the other ingredients, toss, put the lid on and cook on High for 2 hours.

2. Divide the pudding into cups and serve.

Nutrition: calories 213, fat 4, fiber 6, carbs 10, protein 4

Chocolate Cake

Preparation time: 10 minutes

Cooking time: 3 hours

Servings: 10

Ingredients:

- 1 cup flour

- 3 egg whites, whisked

- ½ cup cocoa powder

- ½ cup sugar

- 1 and ½ teaspoons baking powder

- 3 eggs

- 4 tablespoons vegetable oil

- ¾ teaspoon vanilla extract

- 2/3 cup milk

- 1/3 cup dark chocolate chips

Directions:

1. In a bowl, mix sugar with flour, egg whites, cocoa powder, baking powder, milk, oil, eggs, chocolate chips and vanilla extract and whisk really well.

2. Pour this into your lined and greased Slow cooker and cook on Low for 2 hours.

3. Leave the cake aside to cool down, slice and serve.

Nutrition: calories 200, fat 12, fiber 4, carbs 8, protein 6

Chia and Avocado Pudding

Preparation time: 10 minutes

Cooking time: 3 hours

Servings: 2

Ingredients:

- ½ cup almond flour

- 1 tablespoon lime juice

- 2 tablespoons chia seeds

- 1 cup avocado, peeled, pitted and cubed

- 1 teaspoons baking powder

- ¼ teaspoon nutmeg, ground

- ¼ cup almond milk

- 2 tablespoons brown sugar

- 1 egg, whisked

- 2 tablespoons coconut oil, melted

- Cooking spray

Directions:

1. Grease your slow cooker with the cooking spray and mix the chia seeds with the flour, avocado and the other ingredients inside.

2. Put the lid on, cook on High for 3 hours, leave the pudding to cool down, divide into bowls and serve

Nutrition: calories 220, fat 4, fiber 4, carbs 9, protein 6

Berry Cobbler

Preparation time: 10 minutes

Cooking time: 2 hours

Servings: 6

Ingredients:

- 1 pound fresh blackberries

- 1 pound fresh blueberries

- ¾ cup water

- ¾ cup sugar+ 2 tablespoons

- ¾ cup flour

- ¼ cup tapioca flour

- ½ cup arrowroot powder

- 1 teaspoon baking powder

- 2 tablespoons palm sugar

- 1/3 cup milk

- 1 egg, whisked

- 1 teaspoon lemon zest, grated

- 3 tablespoons vegetable oil

Directions:

1. Put blueberries, blackberries, ¾ cup sugar, water and tapioca in your Slow cooker, cover and cook on High for 1 hour.

2. In a bowl, mix flour with arrowroot, the rest of the sugar and baking powder and stir well.

3. In a second bowl, mix the egg with milk, oil and lemon zest.

4. Combine egg mixture with flour mixture, stir well, drop tablespoons of this mix over the berries, cover and cook on High for 1 more hour.

5. Leave cobbler to cool down, divide into dessert bowls and serve.

Nutrition: calories 240, fat 4, fiber 3, carbs 10, protein 6

Almond and Cherries Pudding

Preparation time: 10 minutes

Cooking time: 3 hours

Servings: 2

Ingredients:

- ½ cup almonds, chopped

- ½ cup cherries, pitted and halved

- ½ cup heavy cream

- ½ cup almond milk

- 1 tablespoon butter, soft

- 1 egg

- 2 tablespoons sugar

- ½ cup almond flour

- ½ teaspoon baking powder

- Cooking spray

Directions:

1. Grease the slow cooker with the cooking spray and mix the almonds with the cherries, cream and the other ingredients inside.

2. Put the lid on, cook on High for 3 hours, divide into bowls and serve.

Nutrition: calories 200, fat 4, fiber 2, carbs 8, protein 6

Apple Bread

Preparation time: 10 minutes

Cooking time: 2 hours and 20 minutes

Servings: 6

Ingredients:

- 3 cups apples, cored and cubed

- 1 cup sugar

- 1 tablespoon vanilla extract

- 2 eggs

- 1 tablespoon apple pie spice

- 2 cups flour

- 1 tablespoon baking powder

- 1 tablespoon butter

Directions:

1. In a bowl, mix apples with sugar, vanilla, eggs, apple spice, flour, baking powder and butter, whisk well, pour into your Slow cooker, cover and cook on High for 2 hours and 20 minutes.

2. Leave the bread to cool down, slice and serve.

Nutrition: calories 236, fat 2, fiber 4, carbs 12, protein 4

Vanilla Peach Cream

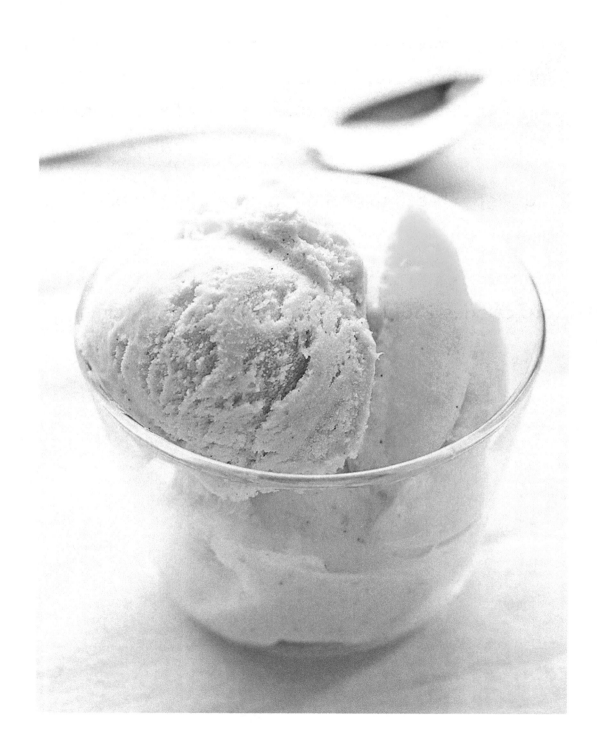

Preparation time: 10 minutes

Cooking time: 3 hours

Servings: 2

Ingredients:

- ¼ teaspoon cinnamon powder

- 1 cup peaches, pitted and chopped

- ¼ cup heavy cream

- Cooking spray

- 1 tablespoon maple syrup

- ½ teaspoons vanilla extract

- 2 tablespoons sugar

Directions:

1. In a blender, mix the peaches with the cinnamon and the other ingredients except the cooking spray and pulse well.

2. Grease the slow cooker with the cooking spray, pour the cream mix inside, put the lid on and cook on Low for 3 hours.

3. Divide the cream into bowls and serve cold.

Nutrition: calories 200, fat 3, fiber 4, carbs 10, protein 9

Banana Cake

Preparation time: 10 minutes

Cooking time: 2 hours

Servings: 6

Ingredients:

- ¾ cup sugar

- 1/3 cup butter, soft

- 1 teaspoon vanilla

- 1 egg

- 3 bananas, mashed

- 1 teaspoon baking powder

- 1 and ½ cups flour

- ½ teaspoons baking soda

- 1/3 cup milk

- Cooking spray

Directions:

1. In a bowl, mix butter with sugar, vanilla extract, eggs, bananas, baking powder, flour, baking soda and milk and whisk.

2. Grease your Slow cooker with the cooking spray, add the batter, spread, cover and cook on High for 2 hours.

3. Leave the cake to cool down, slice and serve.

Nutrition: calories 300, fat 4, fiber 4, carbs 27, protein 4

Cinnamon Plums

Preparation time: 10 minutes

Cooking time: 2 hours

Servings: 2

Ingredients:

- ½ pound plums, pitted and halved

- 2 tablespoons sugar

- 1 teaspoon cinnamon, ground

- ½ cup orange juice

Directions:

1. In your slow cooker, mix the plums with the cinnamon and the other ingredients, toss, put the lid on and cook on Low for 2 hours.

2. Divide into bowls and serve as a dessert.

Nutrition: calories 180, fat 2, fiber 1, carbs 8, protein 8

Chocolate Pudding

Preparation time: 10 minutes

Cooking time: 1 hour

Servings: 4

Ingredients:

- 4 ounces heavy cream

- 4 ounces dark chocolate, cut into chunks

- 1 teaspoon sugar

Directions:

1. In a bowl, mix the cream with chocolate and sugar, whisk well, pour into your slow cooker, cover and cook on High for 1 hour.

2. Divide into bowls and serve cold.

Nutrition: calories 232, fat 12, fiber 6, carbs 9, protein 4

Cardamom Apples

Preparation time: 10 minutes

Cooking time: 2 hours

Servings: 2

Ingredients:

- 1 pound apples, cored and cut into wedges

- ½ cup almond milk

- ¼ teaspoon cardamom, ground

- 2 tablespoons brown sugar

Directions:

1. In your slow cooker, mix the apples with the cardamom and the other ingredients, toss, put the lid on and cook on High for 2 hours.

2. Divide the mix into bowls and serve cold.

Nutrition: calories 280, fat 2, fiber 1, carbs 10, protein 6

Cauliflower Pudding

Preparation time: 5 minutes

Cooking time: 2 hours

Servings: 6

Ingredients:

- 1 tablespoon butter, melted

- 7 ounces cauliflower rice

- 4 ounces water

- 16 ounces milk

- 3 ounces sugar

- 1 egg

- 1 teaspoon cinnamon powder

- 1 teaspoon vanilla extract

Directions:

1. In your Slow cooker, mix butter with cauliflower rice, water, milk, sugar, egg, cinnamon and vanilla extract, stir, cover and cook on High for 2 hours.

2. Divide pudding into bowls and serve cold.

Nutrition: calories 202, fat 2, fiber 6, carbs 18, protein 4

Cherry and Rhubarb Mix

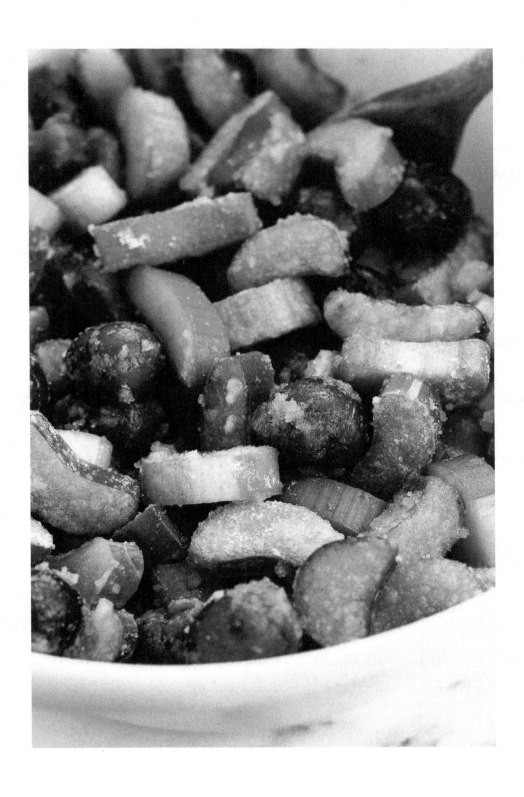

Preparation time: 10 minutes

Cooking time: 2 hours

Servings: 2

Ingredients:

- 2 cups rhubarb, sliced

- ½ cup cherries, pitted

- 1 tablespoon butter, melted

- ¼ cup coconut cream

- ½ cup sugar

Directions:

1. In your slow cooker, mix the rhubarb with the cherries and the other ingredients, toss, put the lid on and cook on High for 2 hours.

2. Divide the mix into bowls and serve cold.

Nutrition: calories 200, fat 2, fiber 3, carbs 6, protein 1

Conclusion

Did you delight in attempting these new and also delightful recipes? sadly we have come to the end of this slow-moving stove recipe book, I truly want it has actually been to your taste. to enhance your health and also wellness we would certainly love to recommend you to incorporate exercise as well as additionally a vibrant method of living together with adhere to these superb meals, so regarding stress the improvements. we will definitely be back quickly with various other dramatically intriguing vegan recipes, a huge hug, see you quickly.

9 781667 138381